HYPOTHYROIDISM JUICING RECIPES COOKBOOK

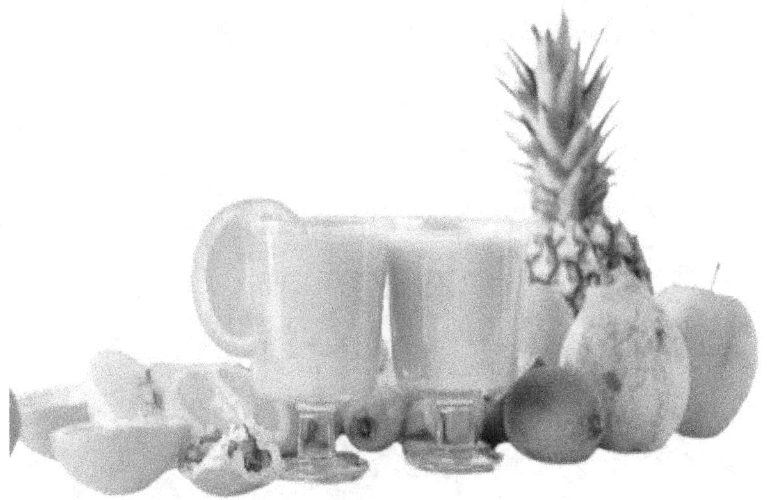

DR. VICKIE STOCK

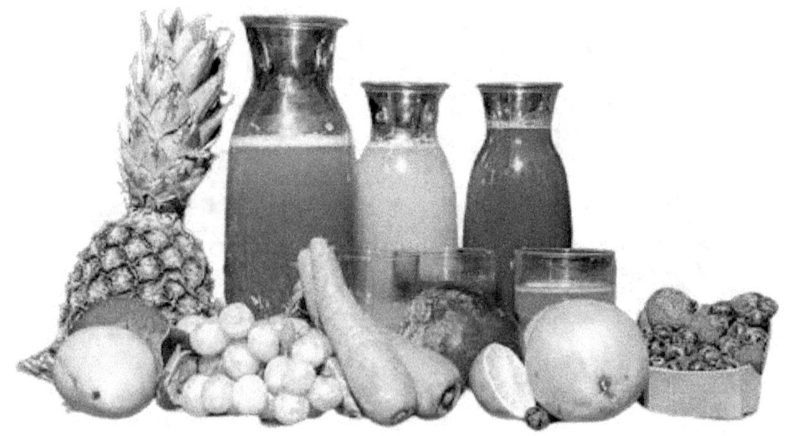

TABLE OF CONTENT

CHAPTER ONE: Introduction

Understanding Hypothyroidism:

Hypothyroidism, often referred to as an underactive thyroid, is a common endocrine disorder characterized by inadequate production of thyroid hormones by the thyroid gland.

These hormones play a crucial role in regulating metabolism, energy production, temperature control, and many other bodily functions. When thyroid hormone levels are low, it can lead to a wide range of symptoms and complications affecting various systems in the body.

Causes:

Autoimmune Thyroiditis (Hashimoto's Thyroiditis): The most common cause of hypothyroidism is autoimmune thyroiditis, an autoimmune condition where the body's immune system attacks the thyroid gland, leading to inflammation and destruction of thyroid tissue.

Thyroid Surgery or Radioactive Iodine Treatment: Removal of the thyroid gland or treatment with radioactive iodine for hyperthyroidism can result in hypothyroidism.

Iodine Deficiency: Inadequate intake of iodine, a crucial mineral required for thyroid hormone synthesis, can lead to hypothyroidism, although this cause is rare in regions where iodine is routinely added to salt or consumed in sufficient quantities through diet.

Medications: Certain medications, such as lithium, amiodarone, and some anti-thyroid drugs, can interfere with thyroid hormone production.

Congenital Hypothyroidism: Some infants are born with an underactive thyroid gland due to genetic defects or abnormal development.

Symptoms: Fatigue, Weight gain, Cold intolerance, Dry skin and hair, Constipation, Muscle weakness, Joint pain, Depression, Memory problems, Menstrual irregularities

Diagnosis:

Diagnosis of hypothyroidism typically involves a combination of medical history, physical examination, and laboratory tests. Blood tests to measure levels of thyroid-stimulating hormone (TSH) and thyroxine (T4) are commonly used to assess thyroid function. Elevated TSH levels and low T4 levels are indicative of hypothyroidism.

Treatment:

Treatment for hypothyroidism usually involves lifelong thyroid hormone replacement therapy with synthetic thyroxine (levothyroxine). The goal of treatment is to restore thyroid hormone levels to normal, alleviate symptoms, and prevent complications.

The dosage of thyroid hormone replacement medication is adjusted based on individual patient response and periodic monitoring of thyroid function tests.

Complications:

Untreated or poorly managed hypothyroidism can lead to various complications, including:

Goiter (enlargement of the thyroid gland)

Cardiovascular problems (high cholesterol, heart disease)

Myxedema (severe hypothyroidism characterized by swelling, lethargy, and decreased mental function)

Infertility and menstrual irregularities

Birth defects in pregnant women with untreated hypothyroidism

Benefits of Juicing for Thyroid Health

Juicing, the process of extracting juices from fruits, vegetables, and herbs, has gained popularity as a convenient and effective way to boost nutrient intake and support overall health.

When it comes to thyroid health, incorporating fresh juices into your diet can offer numerous benefits, helping to optimize thyroid function and alleviate symptoms of hypothyroidism. Below are some of the key benefits of juicing for thyroid health:

1. Nutrient-Rich:

Freshly prepared juices are packed with essential vitamins, minerals, antioxidants, and phytonutrients that are vital for thyroid function and overall health.

Fruits and vegetables such as spinach, kale, carrots, berries, and citrus fruits are particularly rich in nutrients like vitamin C, vitamin A, selenium, iodine, and zinc, which are important for thyroid hormone synthesis, metabolism, and immune function.

2. Supports Detoxification:

Certain vegetables and herbs commonly used in juicing, such as celery, cucumber, parsley, and cilantro, have natural detoxifying properties that help rid the body of toxins and heavy metals that can interfere with thyroid function.

Detoxification supports the liver, which plays a crucial role in converting inactive thyroid hormone (T4) into its active form (T3), thereby promoting optimal thyroid hormone levels.

3. Anti-Inflammatory Effects:

Chronic inflammation is often associated with thyroid disorders, including autoimmune thyroiditis (Hashimoto's thyroiditis). Many fruits and vegetables, especially those with vibrant colors like berries, beets, and turmeric, contain potent anti-inflammatory compounds that can help reduce inflammation in the thyroid gland

CHAPTER TWO: getting started with Juicing

Selecting the Right Ingredients for Thyroid Health Juicing

When it comes to juicing for thyroid health, choosing the right ingredients is crucial to ensure that your juices are nutrient-dense and supportive of thyroid function. Here's a comprehensive guide to selecting the best ingredients for thyroid health juicing:

1. Dark Leafy Greens:

Dark leafy greens such as spinach, kale, Swiss chard, and collard greens are excellent choices for thyroid health juicing. These greens are rich in vitamins A, C, and K, as well as minerals like iron and magnesium. Additionally, they contain antioxidants and chlorophyll, which help reduce inflammation and support detoxification, crucial for thyroid function.

2. Colorful Vegetables:

Incorporate a variety of colorful vegetables into your juices, including carrots, beets, bell peppers, and tomatoes. These vegetables are rich in antioxidants, particularly beta-carotene, which the body converts into vitamin A, essential for thyroid hormone synthesis. Additionally, beets contain nitrates that may improve blood flow to the thyroid gland.

3. Cruciferous Vegetables:

While raw cruciferous vegetables such as broccoli, cabbage, Brussels sprouts, and cauliflower contain compounds called goitrogens, which can interfere with thyroid function when consumed in large amounts, they can still be included in moderation in juices.

Cooking deactivates goitrogens, making them safe for thyroid health. However, if you have thyroid issues, it's best to consult with a healthcare professional before consuming cruciferous vegetables regularly.

4. Berries:

Berries such as blueberries, strawberries, raspberries, and blackberries are rich in antioxidants, particularly vitamin C and flavonoids, which help protect thyroid cells from oxidative stress and inflammation. These fruits also add natural sweetness and vibrant color to your juices.

5. Citrus Fruits:

Citrus fruits like oranges, lemons, and grapefruits are excellent additions to thyroid health juices. They are high in vitamin C, which supports immune function and collagen synthesis. Additionally, citrus fruits add acidity and refreshing flavor to juices, enhancing their taste.

6. Herbs and Spices:

Herbs and spices not only enhance the flavor of your juices but also offer numerous health benefits. Ginger, turmeric, cilantro, parsley, and mint are particularly beneficial for thyroid health. Ginger and turmeric have potent anti-inflammatory properties, while cilantro and parsley support detoxification.

7. Healthy Fats:

Incorporating healthy fats into your juices can help enhance nutrient absorption. Add a small amount of avocado, coconut oil, or nuts/seeds (such as almonds or chia seeds) to your juices to boost their nutritional value and promote satiety.

8. Organic and Fresh Produce:

Whenever possible, choose organic fruits and vegetables to minimize exposure to pesticides and other harmful chemicals. Additionally, use fresh produce to ensure that you're getting the maximum amount of nutrients from your juices.

By selecting the right ingredients and incorporating a variety of nutrient-rich foods into your juices, you can create delicious and nourishing blends that support thyroid health and overall well-being.

Juicing is a popular method for extracting the nutrients from fruits, vegetables, and herbs in a concentrated form. Whether you're new to juicing or a seasoned enthusiast, having the right equipment and techniques can make a significant difference in the quality and efficiency of your juices. Here's a comprehensive guide to juicing equipment and techniques:

1. Juicers:

There are several types of juicers available on the market, each with its own pros and cons:

- ❖ **Centrifugal Juicers:** These juicers work by shredding the fruits and vegetables with a rapidly spinning blade and then extracting the juice through a mesh filter. They are fast and easy to use, making them suitable for beginners. However, they may produce lower-quality juice with less nutrient retention due to heat and oxidation.

- ❖ **Masticating Juicers (Cold Press Juicers):** Masticating juicers operate at a slower speed and use a chewing or grinding mechanism to extract juice from produce. They are more efficient at extracting juice and preserving nutrients, resulting in higher-quality juice with better flavor and shelf life. However, they tend to be more expensive and require more time and effort to clean.

❖ **Twin Gear Juicers:** Twin gear juicers are similar to masticating juicers but use two interlocking gears to crush and press the produce, resulting in even higher juice yields and nutrient retention. They are ideal for juicing hard and fibrous vegetables like kale and wheatgrass but can be more complex to operate and clean.

❖ **Citrus Juicers:** These juicers are designed specifically for juicing citrus fruits like oranges, lemons, and grapefruits. They typically feature a reamer or cone-shaped attachment that extracts the juice when the fruit is pressed onto it.

2. Techniques for Juicing:

❖ Prepare Your Produce: Wash your fruits and vegetables thoroughly before juicing to remove any dirt, pesticides, or contaminants. For fruits with thick skins or pits, such as oranges and peaches, remove the peel and seeds before juicing.

❖ **Cut Produce into Manageable Pieces:** Cut larger fruits and vegetables into smaller pieces that will fit easily into the juicer's feed chute. This helps ensure a smoother juicing process and prevents the juicer from getting clogged.

❖ **Alternate Ingredients:** When juicing a combination of fruits and vegetables, alternate between soft and hard produce to help push the ingredients through the juicer more efficiently. For example, follow leafy greens with cucumber or apple slices.

❖ **Pulp Adjustment:** Most juicers allow you to adjust the pulp level in your juice by changing the settings or using a strainer attachment. Experiment with different pulp levels to find the consistency you prefer.

❖ **Clean Your Juicer Thoroughly:** After juicing, disassemble your juicer and clean each part thoroughly with warm, soapy water to remove any pulp or residue. Some juicers are dishwasher safe, but check the manufacturer's instructions to be sure.

❖ **Drink Fresh:** Freshly made juice is best consumed immediately to maximize nutrient intake and flavor. If you need to store juice for later consumption, store it in an airtight container in the refrigerator for up to 24 hours to minimize nutrient loss.

By choosing the right juicer and mastering the techniques for juicing, you can create delicious and nutritious juices that support your health and well-being. Experiment with different combinations of fruits, vegetables, and herbs to discover your favorite flavor profiles and enjoy the benefits of juicing as part of a healthy lifestyle.

CHAPTER THREE

1: Thyroid-Boosting Green Juice

Ingredients:

- ❖ 2 cups spinach
- ❖ 1 cup kale
- ❖ 1 cucumber
- ❖ 2 celery stalks
- ❖ 1/2 cup parsley
- ❖ 1 lemon, peeled
- ❖ 1-inch piece of ginger

Instructions:

- ❖ Wash all the ingredients thoroughly.
- ❖ Cut the cucumber, celery, and ginger into smaller pieces for easier juicing.
- ❖ Feed all the ingredients through a juicer.
- ❖ Stir the juice well to combine all the flavors.
- ❖ Pour into a glass and enjoy immediately.

Health Benefits:

Spinach and kale are rich in vitamins A, C, and K, as well as minerals like iron and calcium, which support thyroid function.

- ❖ Cucumber and celery provide hydration and are low in calories, making them ideal for weight management, a common concern for individuals with hypothyroidism.
- ❖ Parsley is a good source of antioxidants, including flavonoids and vitamin C, which help reduce inflammation and support immune health.
- ❖ Lemon adds a burst of vitamin C and freshness to the juice, while ginger provides anti-inflammatory properties and aids digestion.

Preparation Time: 10 minutes

2: Immune-Boosting Carrot Juice

Ingredients:

- ❖ 4 carrots, scrubbed and trimmed
- ❖ 2 apples, cored and quartered
- ❖ 1-inch piece of ginger, peeled
- ❖ 1/2 teaspoon ground turmeric
- ❖ 1 lemon, peeled

Instructions:

- ❖ Prepare all the ingredients as directed.
- ❖ Juice the carrots, apples, and ginger together.
- ❖ Stir in the ground turmeric.
- ❖ Juice the lemon separately and add it to the carrot mixture.

❖ Mix well and serve immediately.

Health Benefits:

❖ Carrots are rich in beta-carotene, which is converted into vitamin A in the body and supports immune function.

❖ Apples add natural sweetness and are a good source of fiber, antioxidants, and vitamin C, further boosting immune health.

❖ Ginger and turmeric provide anti-inflammatory properties and help reduce inflammation, a common issue in autoimmune conditions like hypothyroidism.

❖ Lemon adds vitamin C and acidity to the juice, enhancing flavor and providing additional immune support.

Preparation Time: 10 minutes

3: Berry-Beet Antioxidant Blend

Ingredients:

❖ 1 cup mixed berries (such as blueberries, strawberries, raspberries)

❖ 1 small beet, scrubbed and trimmed

❖ 1 orange, peeled

❖ 1 handful spinach

❖ 1 tablespoon chia seeds (optional)

❖ 1 cup coconut water

Instructions:

- ❖ Wash all the berries and spinach thoroughly.
- ❖ Peel the orange and cut the beet into smaller pieces for easier juicing.
- ❖ Juice the berries, beet, orange, and spinach together.
- ❖ Stir in the chia seeds, if using, and let them soak for a few minutes.
- ❖ Add the coconut water to the juice mixture and stir well to combine.
- ❖ Pour into glasses and enjoy immediately.

Health Benefits:

- ❖ Berries are rich in antioxidants, such as anthocyanins and vitamin C, which help protect thyroid cells from oxidative stress and inflammation.
- ❖ Beets are high in nitrates, which support healthy blood flow and may improve thyroid function.
- ❖ Oranges provide vitamin C, essential for immune health and collagen production.
- ❖ Spinach adds additional vitamins, minerals, and fiber, supporting overall health and digestion.
- ❖ Chia seeds are optional but add omega-3 fatty acids and additional fiber, promoting heart health and satiety.

Preparation Time: 10 minutes

Ingredients:

- ❖ 2 large carrots, scrubbed and trimmed
- ❖ 1 apple, cored and quartered
- ❖ 1-inch piece of ginger, peeled
- ❖ 1-inch piece of turmeric, peeled (or 1/2 teaspoon ground turmeric)
- ❖ 1 lemon, peeled
- ❖ 1 tablespoon raw honey (optional)

Instructions:

- ❖ Prepare all the ingredients as directed.
- ❖ Juice the carrots, apple, ginger, and turmeric together.
- ❖ Juice the lemon separately and add it to the carrot mixture.
- ❖ Stir in the raw honey, if using, to sweeten the elixir.
- ❖ Mix well until the honey is dissolved.
- ❖ Pour into glasses and serve immediately.

Health Benefits:

- ❖ Carrots and apples provide vitamins, minerals, and antioxidants that support immune function and thyroid health.

- ❖ Ginger and turmeric have potent anti-inflammatory and antioxidant properties, reducing inflammation and supporting overall well-being.
- ❖ Lemon adds vitamin C and acidity to the elixir, enhancing flavor and providing additional immune support.
- ❖ Raw honey is optional but adds natural sweetness and may provide additional health benefits, including antimicrobial properties.

Preparation Time: 10 minutes

5: Thyroid-Boosting Pineapple Spinach Juice

Ingredients:

- ❖ 2 cups fresh spinach leaves
- ❖ 1 cup chopped pineapple
- ❖ 1 cucumber, peeled and chopped
- ❖ 1-inch piece of ginger, peeled
- ❖ 1 lime, peeled
- ❖ 1 tablespoon fresh mint leaves
- ❖ 1 cup coconut water

Instructions:

- ❖ Wash the spinach leaves thoroughly.
- ❖ Peel and chop the pineapple, cucumber, ginger, and lime.

- ❖ Juice the spinach, pineapple, cucumber, ginger, lime, and mint leaves together.
- ❖ Once juiced, stir in the coconut water until well combined.
- ❖ Pour the juice into glasses and serve immediately.

Health Benefits:

- ❖ Spinach is rich in iron, which is important for thyroid hormone production, and also provides vitamins A and C.
- ❖ Pineapple contains bromelain, an enzyme with anti-inflammatory properties that may help reduce inflammation associated with hypothyroidism.
- ❖ Cucumber is hydrating and low in calories, while ginger provides anti-inflammatory and digestive benefits.
- ❖ Lime adds a citrusy flavor and provides vitamin C, which supports immune function.
- ❖ Mint leaves add freshness and may help soothe digestion.

Preparation Time: 10 minutes

6: Beetroot Carrot Apple Juice

Ingredients:

- ❖ 1 small beetroot, scrubbed and trimmed
- ❖ 2 carrots, scrubbed and trimmed
- ❖ 2 apples, cored and sliced
- ❖ 1-inch piece of ginger, peeled

❖ 1 lemon, peeled

❖ 1 tablespoon raw honey (optional)

❖ 1 cup filtered water

Instructions:

❖ Cut the beetroot, carrots, apples, ginger, and lemon into smaller pieces.

❖ Juice the beetroot, carrots, apples, ginger, and lemon together.

❖ If desired, stir in the raw honey until dissolved.

❖ Dilute the juice with filtered water and mix well.

❖ Pour the juice into glasses and serve immediately over ice, if desired.

Health Benefits:

❖ Beetroot contains nitrates that may improve blood flow and support thyroid function.

❖ Carrots are rich in beta-carotene, which is converted into vitamin A in the body and supports immune function.

❖ Apples add natural sweetness and provide fiber and vitamin C.

❖ Ginger aids digestion and has anti-inflammatory properties.

❖ Lemon adds vitamin C and acidity, enhancing the flavor of the juice.

Preparation Time: 10 minutes

7: Green Thyroid Booster

Ingredients:

- ❖ 2 cups kale leaves
- ❖ 1 cucumber
- ❖ 2 green apples
- ❖ 1/2 lemon, peeled
- ❖ 1-inch piece of ginger
- ❖ 1 tablespoon chia seeds (optional)
- ❖ 1 cup coconut water

Instructions:

- ❖ Wash the kale leaves thoroughly.
- ❖ Peel and chop the cucumber, apples, lemon, and ginger.
- ❖ Juice the kale, cucumber, apples, lemon, and ginger together.
- ❖ If using chia seeds, stir them into the juice and let them soak for a few minutes.
- ❖ Add the coconut water to the juice mixture and stir well to combine.
- ❖ Pour the juice into glasses and enjoy immediately.

Health Benefits:

- ❖ Kale is rich in vitamins A, C, and K, as well as minerals like iron and calcium, which support thyroid function.

- ❖ Cucumber provides hydration and is low in calories, making it ideal for weight management.
- ❖ Green apples add natural sweetness and provide vitamins and antioxidants.
- ❖ Lemon adds a citrusy flavor and provides vitamin C, essential for immune health.
- ❖ Ginger aids digestion and has anti-inflammatory properties.

Preparation Time: 10 minutes

8: Orange Carrot Turmeric Elixir

Ingredients:

- ❖ 3 large carrots, scrubbed and trimmed
- ❖ 2 oranges, peeled
- ❖ 1-inch piece of turmeric, peeled (or 1/2 teaspoon ground turmeric)
- ❖ 1-inch piece of ginger
- ❖ 1 tablespoon raw honey (optional)

Instructions:

- ❖ Prepare all the ingredients as directed.
- ❖ Juice the carrots, oranges, turmeric, and ginger together.
- ❖ If desired, stir in the raw honey until dissolved.
- ❖ Mix well until the honey is fully incorporated.
- ❖ Pour the juice into glasses and serve immediately.

Health Benefits:

- ❖ Carrots are rich in beta-carotene, which is converted into vitamin A in the body and supports immune function.
- ❖ Oranges provide vitamin C, essential for immune health and collagen production.
- ❖ Turmeric and ginger have potent anti-inflammatory properties, reducing inflammation and supporting overall well-being.
- ❖ Raw honey is optional but adds natural sweetness and may provide additional health benefits, including antimicrobial properties.

Preparation Time: 10 minutes

9: Pineapple Ginger Turmeric Delight

Ingredients:

- ❖ 1 cup pineapple chunks
- ❖ 1-inch piece of ginger
- ❖ 1-inch piece of turmeric (or 1/2 teaspoon ground turmeric)
- ❖ 1 orange, peeled
- ❖ 1 carrot, scrubbed and trimmed
- ❖ 1/2 lemon, peeled
- ❖ 1 tablespoon raw honey (optional)
- ❖ 1 cup coconut water

Instructions:

* ❖ Prepare all the ingredients as directed.
* ❖ Juice the pineapple, ginger, turmeric, orange, carrot, and lemon together.
* ❖ If desired, stir in the raw honey until dissolved.
* ❖ Mix well until the honey is fully incorporated.
* ❖ Add the coconut water to the juice mixture and stir well to combine.
* ❖ Pour the juice into glasses and serve immediately.

Health Benefits:

* ❖ Pineapple is rich in bromelain, an enzyme with anti-inflammatory properties that may help reduce inflammation associated with hypothyroidism.
* ❖ Ginger and turmeric provide additional anti-inflammatory benefits and aid digestion.
* ❖ Oranges and carrots are excellent sources of vitamin C and beta-carotene, supporting immune function and thyroid health.
* ❖ Lemon adds acidity and vitamin C to the juice, enhancing flavor and providing additional immune support.
* ❖ Raw honey is optional but adds natural sweetness and may provide antimicrobial benefits.

Preparation Time: 10 minutes

10: Beet Berry Blast

Ingredients:

- ❖ 1 small beet, scrubbed and trimmed
- ❖ 1 cup mixed berries (such as blueberries, strawberries, raspberries)
- ❖ 1 apple, cored and sliced
- ❖ 1-inch piece of ginger
- ❖ 1/2 lemon, peeled
- ❖ 1 tablespoon chia seeds (optional)
- ❖ 1 cup filtered water

Instructions:

- ❖ Wash the beet thoroughly and chop it into smaller pieces.
- ❖ Wash the berries and apple.
- ❖ Peel and chop the ginger and lemon.
- ❖ Juice the beet, berries, apple, ginger, and lemon together.
- ❖ If using chia seeds, stir them into the juice and let them soak for a few minutes.
- ❖ Dilute the juice with filtered water and mix well.
- ❖ Pour the juice into glasses and serve immediately.

Health Benefits:

- ❖ Beets are high in nitrates, which may improve blood flow and support thyroid function.

❖ Berries are rich in antioxidants, protecting thyroid cells from oxidative stress and inflammation.

❖ Apples provide natural sweetness and fiber, supporting digestive health.

❖ Ginger adds a spicy kick and aids digestion.

❖ Lemon adds acidity and vitamin C to the juice, enhancing flavor and providing additional immune support.

❖ Chia seeds are optional but add omega-3 fatty acids and additional fiber, promoting heart health and satiety.

Preparation Time: 10 minutes

11: Kale Pineapple Citrus Cooler

Ingredients:

❖ 2 cups kale leaves

❖ 1 cup pineapple chunks

❖ 1 orange, peeled

❖ 1 lemon, peeled

❖ 1-inch piece of ginger

❖ 1 tablespoon raw honey (optional)

❖ 1 cup coconut water

Instructions:

❖ Wash the kale leaves thoroughly.

❖ Peel and chop the pineapple, orange, lemon, and ginger.

- ❖ Juice the kale, pineapple, orange, lemon, and ginger together.
- ❖ If using raw honey, stir it into the juice until dissolved.
- ❖ Add the coconut water to the juice mixture and stir well to combine.
- ❖ Pour the juice into glasses and serve immediately.

Health Benefits:

- ❖ Kale is rich in vitamins A, C, and K, as well as minerals like iron and calcium, which support thyroid function.
- ❖ Pineapple adds natural sweetness and bromelain, an enzyme with anti-inflammatory properties.
- ❖ Oranges and lemons provide vitamin C, essential for immune health and collagen production.
- ❖ Ginger aids digestion and provides additional anti-inflammatory benefits.
- ❖ Raw honey is optional but adds sweetness and may provide antimicrobial benefits.

Preparation Time: 10 minutes

12: Mango Carrot Turmeric Tonic

Ingredients:

- ❖ 1 ripe mango, peeled and chopped
- ❖ 2 carrots, scrubbed and trimmed

* ❖ 1-inch piece of turmeric (or 1/2 teaspoon ground turmeric)
* ❖ 1/2 lemon, peeled
* ❖ 1-inch piece of ginger
* ❖ 1 tablespoon chia seeds (optional)
* ❖ 1 cup filtered water

Instructions:

* ❖ Wash the carrots and peel the ginger and lemon.
* ❖ Chop the carrots, turmeric, ginger, and lemon into smaller pieces.
* ❖ Juice the mango, carrots, turmeric, ginger, and lemon together.
* ❖ If using chia seeds, stir them into the juice and let them soak for a few minutes.
* ❖ Dilute the juice with filtered water and mix well.
* ❖ Pour the juice into glasses and serve immediately.

Health Benefits:

* ❖ Mango is rich in vitamins A and C, promoting immune health and supporting skin health.
* ❖ Carrots provide beta-carotene, which converts to vitamin A in the body and supports thyroid function.
* ❖ Turmeric and ginger offer anti-inflammatory properties, reducing inflammation and supporting overall well-being.

- ❖ Lemon adds acidity and vitamin C to the juice, enhancing flavor and providing additional immune support.
- ❖ Chia seeds are optional but add omega-3 fatty acids and fiber, promoting heart health and satiety.

Preparation Time: 10 minutes

13: Spinach Beetroot Detox Elixir

Ingredients:

- ❖ 2 cups spinach leaves
- ❖ 1 small beetroot, scrubbed and trimmed
- ❖ 1 green apple, cored and sliced
- ❖ 1 cucumber, peeled and chopped
- ❖ 1-inch piece of ginger
- ❖ 1/2 lemon, peeled
- ❖ 1 tablespoon fresh mint leaves
- ❖ 1 cup coconut water

Instructions:

- ❖ Wash the spinach leaves thoroughly.
- ❖ Chop the beetroot, apple, cucumber, ginger, and lemon into smaller pieces.
- ❖ Juice the spinach, beetroot, apple, cucumber, ginger, lemon, and mint leaves together.
- ❖ Once juiced, stir in the coconut water until well combined.

- ❖ Pour the elixir into glasses and serve immediately.

Health Benefits:

- ❖ Spinach is rich in iron and other essential nutrients that support thyroid health.
- ❖ Beetroot contains nitrates that may improve blood flow and promote overall cardiovascular health.
- ❖ Apples provide natural sweetness and are rich in antioxidants and dietary fiber.
- ❖ Cucumber adds hydration and is low in calories, making it ideal for weight management.
- ❖ Ginger aids digestion and has anti-inflammatory properties, while lemon adds a citrusy kick and vitamin C.
- ❖ Coconut water provides electrolytes and hydration, essential for overall well-being.

Preparation Time: 10 minutes

14: Carrot Orange Ginger Glow

Ingredients:

- ❖ 4 carrots, scrubbed and trimmed
- ❖ 2 oranges, peeled
- ❖ 1-inch piece of ginger
- ❖ 1/2 lemon, peeled
- ❖ 1 tablespoon raw honey (optional)

- ❖ 1 cup filtered water

Instructions:

- ❖ Wash the carrots and peel the ginger and lemon.
- ❖ Chop the carrots, ginger, and lemon into smaller pieces.
- ❖ Juice the carrots, oranges, ginger, and lemon together.
- ❖ If using raw honey, stir it into the juice until dissolved.
- ❖ Dilute the juice with filtered water and mix well.
- ❖ Pour the elixir into glasses and serve immediately.

Health Benefits:

- ❖ Carrots are rich in beta-carotene, which supports immune function and thyroid health.
- ❖ Oranges provide vitamin C, essential for collagen synthesis and immune health.
- ❖ Ginger has anti-inflammatory properties and aids digestion, while lemon adds acidity and vitamin C.
- ❖ Raw honey is optional but adds natural sweetness and may provide antimicrobial benefits.
- ❖ Filtered water helps dilute the juice and promotes hydration, essential for overall well-being.

Preparation Time: 10 minutes

15: Blueberry Kale Antioxidant Blend

Ingredients:

- ❖ 1 cup blueberries
- ❖ 2 cups kale leaves
- ❖ 1 cucumber, peeled and chopped
- ❖ 1 green apple, cored and sliced
- ❖ 1-inch piece of ginger
- ❖ 1/2 lemon, peeled
- ❖ 1 tablespoon chia seeds (optional)
- ❖ 1 cup coconut water

Instructions:

- ❖ Wash the blueberries and kale leaves thoroughly.
- ❖ Peel and chop the cucumber, ginger, and lemon.
- ❖ Juice the blueberries, kale, cucumber, apple, ginger, and lemon together.
- ❖ If using chia seeds, stir them into the juice and let them soak for a few minutes.
- ❖ Add the coconut water to the juice mixture and stir well to combine.
- ❖ Pour the juice into glasses and serve immediately.

Health Benefits:

* Blueberries are rich in antioxidants, which help protect thyroid cells from oxidative stress and inflammation.
* Kale is packed with vitamins A, C, and K, as well as minerals like iron and calcium, which support thyroid function.
* Cucumber provides hydration and is low in calories, making it ideal for weight management.
* Apples add natural sweetness and provide vitamins and antioxidants.
* Ginger aids digestion and has anti-inflammatory properties.
* Lemon adds acidity and vitamin C to the juice, enhancing flavor and providing additional immune support.
* Chia seeds are optional but add omega-3 fatty acids and fiber, promoting heart health and satiety.

Preparation Time: 10 minutes

16: Mango Carrot Turmeric Sunrise

Ingredients:

* 1 ripe mango, peeled and chopped
* 2 carrots, scrubbed and trimmed
* 1-inch piece of turmeric (or 1/2 teaspoon ground turmeric)
* 1/2-inch piece of ginger
* 1/2 lemon, peeled

* 1 tablespoon raw honey (optional)
* 1 cup filtered water

Instructions:

* Wash the carrots and peel the ginger and lemon.
* Chop the carrots, turmeric, ginger, and lemon into smaller pieces.
* Juice the mango, carrots, turmeric, ginger, and lemon together.
* If using raw honey, stir it into the juice until dissolved.
* Dilute the juice with filtered water and mix well.
* Pour the juice into glasses and serve immediately.

Health Benefits:

* Mango is rich in vitamins A and C, promoting immune health and supporting skin health.
* Carrots provide beta-carotene, which converts to vitamin A in the body and supports thyroid function.
* Turmeric and ginger offer anti-inflammatory properties, reducing inflammation and supporting overall well-being.
* Lemon adds acidity and vitamin C to the juice, enhancing flavor and providing additional immune support.
* Raw honey is optional but adds sweetness and may provide antimicrobial benefits.

❖ Filtered water helps dilute the juice and promotes hydration, essential for overall well-being.

Preparation Time: 10 minutes

17: Beet-Apple-Carrot Vitality Juice

Ingredients:

❖ 1 small beet, scrubbed and trimmed

❖ 2 apples, cored and sliced

❖ 2 carrots, scrubbed and trimmed

❖ 1-inch piece of ginger

❖ 1/2 lemon, peeled

❖ 1 tablespoon raw honey (optional)

❖ 1 cup filtered water

Instructions:

❖ Wash the beet, apples, and carrots thoroughly.

❖ Peel the ginger and lemon.

❖ Chop the beet, apples, carrots, ginger, and lemon into smaller pieces.

❖ Juice the beet, apples, carrots, ginger, and lemon together.

❖ If using raw honey, stir it into the juice until dissolved.

❖ Dilute the juice with filtered water and mix well.

❖ Pour the juice into glasses and serve immediately.

Health Benefits:

- ❖ Beets are high in nitrates, which may improve blood flow and support thyroid function.
- ❖ Apples provide natural sweetness and are rich in antioxidants and dietary fiber.
- ❖ Carrots are a good source of beta-carotene, which supports immune function and thyroid health.
- ❖ Ginger aids digestion and provides anti-inflammatory benefits.
- ❖ Lemon adds acidity and vitamin C to the juice, enhancing flavor and providing additional immune support.
- ❖ Raw honey is optional but adds sweetness and may provide antimicrobial benefits.
- ❖ Filtered water helps dilute the juice and promotes hydration, essential for overall well-being.

Preparation Time: 10 minutes

18: Pineapple-Turmeric-Cucumber Refresh

Ingredients:

- ❖ 1 cup pineapple chunks
- ❖ 1 cucumber, peeled and chopped
- ❖ 1-inch piece of turmeric (or 1/2 teaspoon ground turmeric)
- ❖ 1/2 lemon, peeled

- ❖ 1 tablespoon fresh mint leaves

- ❖ 1 cup coconut water

- ❖ Ice cubes (optional)

Instructions:

- ❖ Wash the cucumber and lemon thoroughly.

- ❖ Peel the cucumber and lemon.

- ❖ Chop the pineapple, cucumber, turmeric, and lemon into smaller pieces.

- ❖ Juice the pineapple, cucumber, turmeric, and lemon together.

- ❖ Stir in the fresh mint leaves.

- ❖ Add the coconut water and mix well.

- ❖ Pour the juice into glasses over ice cubes, if desired, and serve immediately.

Health Benefits:

- ❖ Pineapple contains bromelain, an enzyme with anti-inflammatory properties.

- ❖ Cucumber provides hydration and is low in calories, making it ideal for weight management.

- ❖ Turmeric offers anti-inflammatory benefits and supports overall well-being.

- ❖ Lemon adds acidity and vitamin C to the juice, enhancing flavor and providing additional immune support.

❖ Fresh mint leaves add a refreshing touch to the juice.

❖ Coconut water provides electrolytes and hydration, essential for overall well-being.

Preparation Time: 10 minutes

19: Green Citrus Energy Boost

Ingredients:

❖ 2 cups spinach leaves

❖ 1 cucumber, peeled and chopped

❖ 2 green apples, cored and sliced

❖ 1-inch piece of ginger

❖ 1/2 lemon, peeled

❖ 1 tablespoon chia seeds (optional)

❖ 1 cup coconut water

Instructions:

❖ Wash the spinach leaves thoroughly.

❖ Chop the cucumber, apples, ginger, and lemon into smaller pieces.

❖ Juice the spinach, cucumber, apples, ginger, and lemon together.

❖ If using chia seeds, stir them into the juice and let them soak for a few minutes.

- ❖ Add the coconut water to the juice mixture and stir well to combine.
- ❖ Pour the juice into glasses and serve immediately.

Health Benefits:

- ❖ Spinach is rich in iron and other essential nutrients that support thyroid health.
- ❖ Cucumber provides hydration and is low in calories, making it ideal for weight management.
- ❖ Green apples add natural sweetness and are a good source of vitamins and antioxidants.
- ❖ Ginger aids digestion and has anti-inflammatory properties.
- ❖ Lemon adds acidity and vitamin C to the juice, enhancing flavor and providing additional immune support.
- ❖ Chia seeds are optional but add omega-3 fatty acids and fiber, promoting heart health and satiety.
- ❖ Coconut water provides electrolytes and hydration, essential for overall well-being.

Preparation Time: 10 minutes

20: Orange Carrot Turmeric Glow

Ingredients:

- ❖ 4 carrots, scrubbed and trimmed
- ❖ 2 oranges, peeled

- ❖ 1-inch piece of turmeric (or 1/2 teaspoon ground turmeric)
- ❖ 1/2 lemon, peeled
- ❖ 1 tablespoon raw honey (optional)
- ❖ 1 cup filtered water

Instructions:

- ❖ Wash the carrots and peel the turmeric and lemon.
- ❖ Chop the carrots, turmeric, and lemon into smaller pieces.
- ❖ Juice the carrots, oranges, turmeric, and lemon together.
- ❖ If using raw honey, stir it into the juice until dissolved.
- ❖ Dilute the juice with filtered water and mix well.
- ❖ Pour the juice into glasses and serve immediately.

Health Benefits:

- ❖ Carrots are rich in beta-carotene, which supports immune function and thyroid health.
- ❖ Oranges provide vitamin C, essential for collagen synthesis and immune health.
- ❖ Turmeric offers anti-inflammatory benefits and supports overall well-being.
- ❖ Lemon adds acidity and vitamin C to the juice, enhancing flavor and providing additional immune support.
- ❖ Raw honey is optional but adds sweetness and may provide antimicrobial benefits.

❖ Filtered water helps dilute the juice and promotes hydration, essential for overall well-being.

Preparation Time: 10 minutes

21: Berry Beetroot Blast

Ingredients:

- ❖ 1 cup mixed berries (such as blueberries, raspberries, strawberries)
- ❖ 1 small beetroot, scrubbed and trimmed
- ❖ 1 cucumber, peeled and chopped
- ❖ 1-inch piece of ginger
- ❖ 1/2 lemon, peeled
- ❖ 1 tablespoon raw honey (optional)
- ❖ 1 cup coconut water

Instructions:

- ❖ Wash the berries and beetroot thoroughly.
- ❖ Peel the ginger and lemon.
- ❖ Chop the beetroot, cucumber, ginger, and lemon into smaller pieces.
- ❖ Juice the berries, beetroot, cucumber, ginger, and lemon together.
- ❖ If using raw honey, stir it into the juice until dissolved.

- ❖ Add the coconut water to the juice mixture and stir well to combine.
- ❖ Pour the juice into glasses and serve immediately.

Health Benefits:

- ❖ Berries are rich in antioxidants, which help protect thyroid cells from oxidative stress and inflammation.
- ❖ Beetroot contains nitrates that may improve blood flow and support thyroid function.
- ❖ Cucumber provides hydration and is low in calories, making it ideal for weight management.
- ❖ Ginger aids digestion and provides anti-inflammatory benefits.
- ❖ Lemon adds acidity and vitamin C to the juice, enhancing flavor and providing additional immune support.
- ❖ Raw honey is optional but adds sweetness and may provide antimicrobial benefits.
- ❖ Coconut water provides electrolytes and hydration, essential for overall well-being.

Preparation Time: 10 minutes

22: Spinach Pineapple Ginger Zing

Ingredients:

- ❖ 2 cups spinach leaves

- ❖ 1 cup pineapple chunks

- ❖ 1 cucumber, peeled and chopped

- ❖ 1-inch piece of ginger

- ❖ 1/2 lemon, peeled

- ❖ 1 tablespoon chia seeds (optional)

- ❖ 1 cup coconut water

Instructions:

- ❖ Wash the spinach leaves thoroughly.

- ❖ Peel the ginger and lemon.

- ❖ Chop the pineapple, cucumber, ginger, and lemon into smaller pieces.

- ❖ Juice the spinach, pineapple, cucumber, ginger, and lemon together.

- ❖ If using chia seeds, stir them into the juice and let them soak for a few minutes.

- ❖ Add the coconut water to the juice mixture and stir well to combine.

- ❖ Pour the juice into glasses and serve immediately.

Health Benefits:

- ❖ Spinach is rich in iron and other essential nutrients that support thyroid health.

- ❖ Pineapple contains bromelain, an enzyme with anti-inflammatory properties.

- ❖ Cucumber provides hydration and is low in calories, making it ideal for weight management.
- ❖ Ginger aids digestion and provides anti-inflammatory benefits.
- ❖ Lemon adds acidity and vitamin C to the juice, enhancing flavor and providing additional immune support.
- ❖ Chia seeds are optional but add omega-3 fatty acids and fiber, promoting heart health and satiety.
- ❖ Coconut water provides electrolytes and hydration, essential for overall well-being.

Preparation Time: 10 minutes

23: Carrot-Apple-Ginger Elixir

Ingredients:

- ❖ 4 carrots, scrubbed and trimmed
- ❖ 2 apples, cored and sliced
- ❖ 1-inch piece of ginger
- ❖ 1/2 lemon, peeled
- ❖ 1 tablespoon raw honey (optional)
- ❖ 1 cup filtered water

Instructions:

- ❖ Wash the carrots and peel the ginger and lemon.

- ❖ Chop the carrots, apples, ginger, and lemon into smaller pieces.
- ❖ Juice the carrots, apples, ginger, and lemon together.
- ❖ If using raw honey, stir it into the juice until dissolved.
- ❖ Dilute the juice with filtered water and mix well.
- ❖ Pour the elixir into glasses and serve immediately.

Health Benefits:

- ❖ Carrots are rich in beta-carotene, which supports immune function and thyroid health.
- ❖ Apples provide natural sweetness and are rich in antioxidants and dietary fiber.
- ❖ Ginger aids digestion and provides anti-inflammatory benefits.
- ❖ Lemon adds acidity and vitamin C to the juice, enhancing flavor and providing additional immune support.
- ❖ Raw honey is optional but adds sweetness and may provide antimicrobial benefits.
- ❖ Filtered water helps dilute the juice and promotes hydration, essential for overall well-being.

Preparation Time: 10 minutes

24: Spinach-Orange-Turmeric Delight

Ingredients:

- ❖ 2 cups spinach leaves
- ❖ 2 oranges, peeled
- ❖ 1-inch piece of turmeric (or 1/2 teaspoon ground turmeric)
- ❖ 1/2 lemon, peeled
- ❖ 1 tablespoon fresh mint leaves
- ❖ 1 cup coconut water

Instructions:

- ❖ Wash the spinach leaves thoroughly.
- ❖ Peel the turmeric, lemon, and oranges.
- ❖ Chop the oranges into smaller pieces.
- ❖ Juice the spinach, oranges, turmeric, and lemon together.
- ❖ Stir in the fresh mint leaves.
- ❖ Add the coconut water and mix well.
- ❖ Pour the juice into glasses and serve immediately.

Health Benefits:

- ❖ Spinach is rich in iron and other essential nutrients that support thyroid health.
- ❖ Oranges provide vitamin C, essential for collagen synthesis and immune health.

- ❖ Turmeric offers anti-inflammatory benefits and supports overall well-being.
- ❖ Lemon adds acidity and vitamin C to the juice, enhancing flavor and providing additional immune support.
- ❖ Fresh mint leaves add a refreshing touch to the juice.
- ❖ Coconut water provides electrolytes and hydration, essential for overall well-being.

Preparation Time: 10 minutes

25: Berry Spinach Revitalizer

Ingredients:

- 1 cup mixed berries (such as blueberries, raspberries, strawberries)
- 2 cups spinach leaves
- 1 cucumber, peeled and chopped
- 1-inch piece of ginger
- 1/2 lemon, peeled
- 1 tablespoon raw honey (optional)
- 1 cup coconut water

Instructions:

- Wash the berries and spinach leaves thoroughly.
- Peel the ginger and lemon.
- Chop the cucumber, ginger, and lemon into smaller pieces.

- Juice the berries, spinach, cucumber, ginger, and lemon together.
- If using raw honey, stir it into the juice until dissolved.
- Add the coconut water to the juice mixture and stir well to combine.
- Pour the juice into glasses and serve immediately.

Health Benefits:

- Berries are rich in antioxidants, which help protect thyroid cells from oxidative stress and inflammation.
- Spinach is packed with vitamins and minerals that support thyroid health.
- Cucumber provides hydration and is low in calories, making it ideal for weight management.
- Ginger aids digestion and provides anti-inflammatory benefits.
- Lemon adds acidity and vitamin C to the juice, enhancing flavor and providing additional immune support.
- Raw honey is optional but adds sweetness and may provide antimicrobial benefits.
- Coconut water provides electrolytes and hydration, essential for overall well-being.

Preparation Time: 10 minutes

Ingredients:

- 1 cup pineapple chunks
- 1 ripe mango, peeled and chopped
- 1-inch piece of turmeric (or 1/2 teaspoon ground turmeric)
- 1/2 lemon, peeled
- 1 tablespoon fresh mint leaves
- 1 cup coconut water

Instructions:

- Peel the turmeric and lemon.
- Chop the pineapple, mango, turmeric, and lemon into smaller pieces.
- Juice the pineapple, mango, turmeric, and lemon together.
- Stir in the fresh mint leaves.
- Add the coconut water and mix well.
- Pour the juice into glasses and serve immediately.

Health Benefits:

- Pineapple and mango add natural sweetness and are rich in vitamins and antioxidants.
- Turmeric offers anti-inflammatory benefits and supports overall well-being.

- Lemon adds acidity and vitamin C to the juice, enhancing flavor and providing additional immune support.
- Fresh mint leaves add a refreshing touch to the juice.
- Coconut water provides electrolytes and hydration, essential for overall well-being.

Preparation Time: 10 minutes

27: Kiwi Kale Cleanse

Ingredients:

- 2 kiwis, peeled and chopped
- 2 cups kale leaves
- 1 cucumber, peeled and chopped
- 1-inch piece of ginger
- 1/2 lemon, peeled
- 1 tablespoon chia seeds (optional)
- 1 cup coconut water

Instructions:

- Wash the kale leaves thoroughly.
- Peel the ginger and lemon.
- Chop the cucumber, ginger, and lemon into smaller pieces.
- Juice the kiwis, kale, cucumber, ginger, and lemon together.

- If using chia seeds, stir them into the juice and let them soak for a few minutes.
- Add the coconut water to the juice mixture and stir well to combine.
- Pour the juice into glasses and serve immediately.

Health Benefits:

- Kiwis are rich in vitamin C and fiber, which support immune function and digestion.
- Kale is packed with vitamins and minerals that support thyroid health.
- Cucumber provides hydration and is low in calories, making it ideal for weight management.
- Ginger aids digestion and provides anti-inflammatory benefits.
- Lemon adds acidity and vitamin C to the juice, enhancing flavor and providing additional immune support.
- Chia seeds are optional but add omega-3 fatty acids and fiber, promoting heart health and satiety.
- Coconut water provides electrolytes and hydration, essential for overall well-being.

Preparation Time: 10 minutes

28: Peach Spinach Refresher

Ingredients:

- 2 peaches, pitted and chopped
- 2 cups spinach leaves
- 1 cucumber, peeled and chopped
- 1-inch piece of ginger
- 1/2 lemon, peeled
- 1 tablespoon raw honey (optional)
- 1 cup coconut water

Instructions:

- Wash the spinach leaves thoroughly.
- Peel the ginger and lemon.
- Chop the peaches, cucumber, ginger, and lemon into smaller pieces.
- Juice the peaches, spinach, cucumber, ginger, and lemon together.
- If using raw honey, stir it into the juice until dissolved.
- Add the coconut water to the juice mixture and stir well to combine.
- Pour the juice into glasses and serve immediately.

Health Benefits:

- Peaches add natural sweetness and are rich in vitamins A and C, promoting immune health and supporting skin health.
- Spinach is packed with vitamins and minerals that support thyroid health.
- Cucumber provides hydration and is low in calories, making it ideal for weight management.
- Ginger aids digestion and provides anti-inflammatory benefits.
- Lemon adds acidity and vitamin C to the juice, enhancing flavor and providing additional immune support.
- Raw honey is optional but adds sweetness and may provide antimicrobial benefits.
- Coconut water provides electrolytes and hydration, essential for overall well-being.

Preparation Time: 10 minutes

29: Mango Spinach Sunshine

Ingredients:

- 1 ripe mango, peeled and chopped
- 2 cups spinach leaves
- 1 cucumber, peeled and chopped
- 1-inch piece of ginger

- 1/2 lemon, peeled

- 1 tablespoon raw honey (optional)

- 1 cup coconut water

Instructions:

- Wash the spinach leaves thoroughly.

- Peel the ginger and lemon.

- Chop the mango, cucumber, ginger, and lemon into smaller pieces.

- Juice the mango, spinach, cucumber, ginger, and lemon together.

- If using raw honey, stir it into the juice until dissolved.

- Add the coconut water to the juice mixture and stir well to combine.

- Pour the juice into glasses and serve immediately.

Health Benefits:

- Mangoes are rich in vitamins A and C, which support immune health and promote skin health.

- Spinach is packed with vitamins and minerals that support thyroid health.

- Cucumber provides hydration and is low in calories, making it ideal for weight management.

- Ginger aids digestion and provides anti-inflammatory benefits.
- Lemon adds acidity and vitamin C to the juice, enhancing flavor and providing additional immune support.
- Raw honey is optional but adds sweetness and may provide antimicrobial benefits.
- Coconut water provides electrolytes and hydration, essential for overall well-being.

Preparation Time: 10 minutes

30: Pineapple Beetroot Detoxifier

Ingredients:

- 1 cup pineapple chunks
- 1 small beetroot, scrubbed and trimmed
- 1 cucumber, peeled and chopped
- 1-inch piece of ginger
- 1/2 lemon, peeled
- 1 tablespoon chia seeds (optional)
- 1 cup coconut water

Instructions:

- Wash the beetroot and peel the ginger and lemon.
- Chop the pineapple, beetroot, cucumber, ginger, and lemon into smaller pieces.

- Juice the pineapple, beetroot, cucumber, ginger, and lemon together.
- If using chia seeds, stir them into the juice and let them soak for a few minutes.
- Add the coconut water to the juice mixture and stir well to combine.
- Pour the juice into glasses and serve immediately.

Health Benefits:

- Pineapple contains bromelain, an enzyme with anti-inflammatory properties.
- Beetroot is rich in nitrates, which may improve blood flow and support thyroid function.
- Cucumber provides hydration and is low in calories, making it ideal for weight management.
- Ginger aids digestion and provides anti-inflammatory benefits.
- Lemon adds acidity and vitamin C to the juice, enhancing flavor and providing additional immune support.
- Chia seeds are optional but add omega-3 fatty acids and fiber, promoting heart health and satiety.
- Coconut water provides electrolytes and hydration, essential for overall well-being.

Preparation Time: 10 minutes

31: Green Apple Spinach Refresher

Ingredients:

- ❖ 2 green apples, cored and sliced
- ❖ 2 cups spinach leaves
- ❖ 1 cucumber, peeled and chopped
- ❖ 1-inch piece of ginger
- ❖ 1/2 lemon, peeled
- ❖ 1 tablespoon raw honey (optional)
- ❖ 1 cup coconut water

Instructions:

- ❖ Wash the spinach leaves thoroughly.
- ❖ Peel the ginger and lemon.
- ❖ Chop the apples, cucumber, ginger, and lemon into smaller pieces.
- ❖ Juice the apples, spinach, cucumber, ginger, and lemon together.
- ❖ If using raw honey, stir it into the juice until dissolved.
- ❖ Add the coconut water to the juice mixture and stir well to combine.
- ❖ Pour the juice into glasses and serve immediately.

Health Benefits:

- Green apples add natural sweetness and are rich in vitamins and antioxidants.
- Spinach is packed with vitamins and minerals that support thyroid health.
- Cucumber provides hydration and is low in calories, making it ideal for weight management.
- Ginger aids digestion and provides anti-inflammatory benefits.
- Lemon adds acidity and vitamin C to the juice, enhancing flavor and providing additional immune support.
- Raw honey is optional but adds sweetness and may provide antimicrobial benefits.
- Coconut water provides electrolytes and hydration, essential for overall well-being.

Preparation Time: 10 minutes

32: Orange Carrot Turmeric Elixir

Ingredients:

- 4 carrots, scrubbed and trimmed
- 2 oranges, peeled
- 1-inch piece of turmeric (or 1/2 teaspoon ground turmeric)
- 1/2 lemon, peeled

- ❖ 1 tablespoon fresh mint leaves
- ❖ 1 cup coconut water

Instructions:

- ❖ Peel the turmeric and lemon.
- ❖ Chop the carrots and oranges into smaller pieces.
- ❖ Juice the carrots, oranges, turmeric, and lemon together.
- ❖ Stir in the fresh mint leaves.
- ❖ Add the coconut water and mix well.
- ❖ Pour the elixir into glasses and serve immediately.

Health Benefits:

- ❖ Carrots are rich in beta-carotene, which supports immune function and thyroid health.
- ❖ Oranges provide vitamin C, essential for collagen synthesis and immune health.
- ❖ Turmeric offers anti-inflammatory benefits and supports overall well-being.
- ❖ Lemon adds acidity and vitamin C to the juice, enhancing flavor and providing additional immune support.
- ❖ Fresh mint leaves add a refreshing touch to the juice.
- ❖ Coconut water provides electrolytes and hydration, essential for overall well-being.

Preparation Time: 10 minutes

Ingredients:

- 1 cup mixed berries (such as blueberries, raspberries, strawberries)
- 1 cucumber, peeled and chopped
- 2 celery stalks, chopped
- 1-inch piece of ginger
- 1/2 lemon, peeled
- 1 tablespoon chia seeds (optional)
- 1 cup coconut water

Instructions:

- Wash the berries, cucumber, and celery thoroughly.
- Peel the ginger and lemon.
- Chop the cucumber, celery, ginger, and lemon into smaller pieces.
- Juice the berries, cucumber, celery, ginger, and lemon together.
- If using chia seeds, stir them into the juice and let them soak for a few minutes.
- Add the coconut water to the juice mixture and stir well to combine.
- Pour the juice into glasses and serve immediately.

Health Benefits:

- ❖ Berries are rich in antioxidants, which help protect thyroid cells from oxidative stress and inflammation.
- ❖ Cucumber provides hydration and is low in calories, making it ideal for weight management.
- ❖ Celery is rich in vitamins and minerals, including vitamin K, potassium, and folate.
- ❖ Ginger aids digestion and provides anti-inflammatory benefits.
- ❖ Lemon adds acidity and vitamin C to the juice, enhancing flavor and providing additional immune support.
- ❖ Chia seeds are optional but add omega-3 fatty acids and fiber, promoting heart health and satiety.
- ❖ Coconut water provides electrolytes and hydration, essential for overall well-being.

Preparation Time: 10 minutes

34: Pineapple Mint Cooler

Ingredients:

- ❖ 1 cup pineapple chunks
- ❖ 1 cucumber, peeled and chopped
- ❖ 1 handful of fresh mint leaves
- ❖ 1-inch piece of ginger

❖ 1/2 lemon, peeled

❖ 1 tablespoon raw honey (optional)

❖ 1 cup coconut water

Instructions:

❖ Wash the mint leaves thoroughly.

❖ Peel the ginger and lemon.

❖ Chop the pineapple, cucumber, ginger, and lemon into smaller pieces.

❖ Juice the pineapple, cucumber, ginger, and lemon together.

❖ Blend the fresh mint leaves with a little water to make a mint paste.

❖ Mix the mint paste into the juice.

❖ If using raw honey, stir it into the juice until dissolved.

❖ Add the coconut water to the juice mixture and stir well to combine.

❖ Pour the juice into glasses and serve immediately.

Health Benefits:

❖ Pineapple contains bromelain, an enzyme with anti-inflammatory properties.

❖ Cucumber provides hydration and is low in calories, making it ideal for weight management.

❖ Fresh mint leaves add a refreshing taste and may aid digestion.

- ❖ Ginger provides anti-inflammatory benefits and aids digestion.
- ❖ Lemon adds acidity and vitamin C to the juice, enhancing flavor and providing additional immune support.
- ❖ Raw honey is optional but adds sweetness and may provide antimicrobial benefits.
- ❖ Coconut water provides electrolytes and hydration, essential for overall well-being.

Preparation Time: 10 minutes

35: Kale Pineapple Paradise

Ingredients:

- ❖ 2 cups kale leaves
- ❖ 1 cup pineapple chunks
- ❖ 1 cucumber, peeled and chopped
- ❖ 1-inch piece of ginger
- ❖ 1/2 lemon, peeled
- ❖ 1 tablespoon raw honey (optional)
- ❖ 1 cup coconut water

Instructions:

- ❖ Wash the kale leaves thoroughly.
- ❖ Peel the ginger and lemon.

- ❖ Chop the pineapple, cucumber, ginger, and lemon into smaller pieces.
- ❖ Juice the kale, pineapple, cucumber, ginger, and lemon together.
- ❖ If using raw honey, stir it into the juice until dissolved.
- ❖ Add the coconut water to the juice mixture and stir well to combine.
- ❖ Pour the juice into glasses and serve immediately.

Health Benefits:

- ❖ Kale is rich in vitamins and minerals, including vitamins A, C, and K, which support thyroid health.
- ❖ Pineapple contains bromelain, an enzyme with anti-inflammatory properties.
- ❖ Cucumber provides hydration and is low in calories, making it ideal for weight management.
- ❖ Ginger aids digestion and provides anti-inflammatory benefits.
- ❖ Lemon adds acidity and vitamin C to the juice, enhancing flavor and providing additional immune support.
- ❖ Raw honey is optional but adds sweetness and may provide antimicrobial benefits.
- ❖ Coconut water provides electrolytes and hydration, essential for overall well-being.

Preparation Time: 10 minutes

36: Blueberry Beetroot Bliss

Ingredients:

- ❖ 1 cup blueberries
- ❖ 1 small beetroot, scrubbed and trimmed
- ❖ 1 cucumber, peeled and chopped
- ❖ 1-inch piece of ginger
- ❖ 1/2 lemon, peeled
- ❖ 1 tablespoon chia seeds (optional)
- ❖ 1 cup coconut water

Instructions:

- ❖ Wash the blueberries and beetroot thoroughly.
- ❖ Peel the ginger and lemon.
- ❖ Chop the beetroot, cucumber, ginger, and lemon into smaller pieces.
- ❖ Juice the blueberries, beetroot, cucumber, ginger, and lemon together.
- ❖ If using chia seeds, stir them into the juice and let them soak for a few minutes.
- ❖ Add the coconut water to the juice mixture and stir well to combine.
- ❖ Pour the juice into glasses and serve immediately.

Health Benefits:

- ❖ Blueberries are rich in antioxidants, which help protect thyroid cells from oxidative stress and inflammation.
- ❖ Beetroot is high in nitrates, which may improve blood flow and support thyroid function.
- ❖ Cucumber provides hydration and is low in calories, making it ideal for weight management.
- ❖ Ginger aids digestion and provides anti-inflammatory benefits.
- ❖ Lemon adds acidity and vitamin C to the juice, enhancing flavor and providing additional immune support.
- ❖ Chia seeds are optional but add omega-3 fatty acids and fiber, promoting heart health and satiety.
- ❖ Coconut water provides electrolytes and hydration, essential for overall well-being.

Preparation Time: 10 minutes

37: Spinach Apple Detoxifier

Ingredients:

- ❖ 2 cups spinach leaves
- ❖ 2 apples, cored and sliced
- ❖ 1 cucumber, peeled and chopped
- ❖ 1-inch piece of ginger

*   1/2 lemon, peeled

*   1 tablespoon raw honey (optional)

*   1 cup coconut water

Instructions:

*   Wash the spinach leaves thoroughly.

*   Peel the ginger and lemon.

*   Chop the apples, cucumber, ginger, and lemon into smaller pieces.

*   Juice the spinach, apples, cucumber, ginger, and lemon together.

*   If using raw honey, stir it into the juice until dissolved.

*   Add the coconut water to the juice mixture and stir well to combine.

*   Pour the juice into glasses and serve immediately.

Health Benefits:

*   Spinach is packed with vitamins and minerals that support thyroid health.

*   Apples provide natural sweetness and are rich in antioxidants and dietary fiber.

*   Cucumber provides hydration and is low in calories, making it ideal for weight management.

*   Ginger aids digestion and provides anti-inflammatory benefits.

- Lemon adds acidity and vitamin C to the juice, enhancing flavor and providing additional immune support.
- Raw honey is optional but adds sweetness and may provide antimicrobial benefits.
- Coconut water provides electrolytes and hydration, essential for overall well-being.

Preparation Time: 10 minutes

38: Orange Carrot Ginger Zing

Ingredients:

- 4 carrots, scrubbed and trimmed
- 2 oranges, peeled
- 1-inch piece of ginger
- 1/2 lemon, peeled
- 1 tablespoon fresh mint leaves
- 1 cup coconut water

Instructions:

- Peel the ginger and lemon.
- Chop the carrots and oranges into smaller pieces.
- Juice the carrots, oranges, ginger, and lemon together.
- Stir in the fresh mint leaves.
- Add the coconut water and mix well.
- Pour the juice into glasses and serve immediately.

Health Benefits:

- ❖ Carrots are rich in beta-carotene, which supports immune function and thyroid health.
- ❖ Oranges provide vitamin C, essential for collagen synthesis and immune health.
- ❖ Ginger offers anti-inflammatory benefits and aids digestion.
- ❖ Lemon adds acidity and vitamin C to the juice, enhancing flavor and providing additional immune support.
- ❖ Fresh mint leaves add a refreshing taste and may aid digestion.
- ❖ Coconut water provides electrolytes and hydration, essential for overall well-being.

Preparation Time: 10 minutes

39: Beetroot Berry Blast

Ingredients:

- ❖ 1 small beetroot, scrubbed and trimmed
- ❖ 1 cup mixed berries (such as blueberries, raspberries, strawberries)
- ❖ 1 cucumber, peeled and chopped
- ❖ 1-inch piece of ginger
- ❖ 1/2 lemon, peeled
- ❖ 1 tablespoon chia seeds (optional)

❖ 1 cup coconut water

Instructions:

❖ Wash the beetroot and berries thoroughly.

❖ Peel the ginger and lemon.

❖ Chop the beetroot, cucumber, ginger, and lemon into smaller pieces.

❖ Juice the beetroot, berries, cucumber, ginger, and lemon together.

❖ If using chia seeds, stir them into the juice and let them soak for a few minutes.

❖ Add the coconut water to the juice mixture and stir well to combine.

❖ Pour the juice into glasses and serve immediately.

Health Benefits:

❖ Beetroot is high in nitrates, which may improve blood flow and support thyroid function.

❖ Berries are rich in antioxidants, which help protect thyroid cells from oxidative stress and inflammation.

❖ Cucumber provides hydration and is low in calories, making it ideal for weight management.

❖ Ginger aids digestion and provides anti-inflammatory benefits.

* Lemon adds acidity and vitamin C to the juice, enhancing flavor and providing additional immune support.
* Chia seeds are optional but add omega-3 fatty acids and fiber, promoting heart health and satiety.
* Coconut water provides electrolytes and hydration, essential for overall well-being.

Preparation Time: 10 minutes

40: Turmeric Citrus Cleanse

Ingredients:

* 2 oranges, peeled
* 1 grapefruit, peeled
* 1-inch piece of turmeric (or 1/2 teaspoon ground turmeric)
* 1/2 lemon, peeled
* 1 tablespoon raw honey (optional)
* 1 cup coconut water

Instructions:

* Peel the turmeric and lemon.
* Chop the oranges, grapefruit, turmeric, and lemon into smaller pieces.
* Juice the oranges, grapefruit, turmeric, and lemon together.
* If using raw honey, stir it into the juice until dissolved.

- ❖ Add the coconut water to the juice mixture and stir well to combine.
- ❖ Pour the juice into glasses and serve immediately.

Health Benefits:

- ❖ Oranges and grapefruits provide vitamin C, essential for collagen synthesis and immune health.
- ❖ Turmeric offers anti-inflammatory benefits and supports overall well-being.
- ❖ Lemon adds acidity and vitamin C to the juice, enhancing flavor and providing additional immune support.
- ❖ Raw honey is optional but adds sweetness and may provide antimicrobial benefits.
- ❖ Coconut water provides electrolytes and hydration, essential for overall well-being.

Preparation Time: 10 minutes

CONCLUSION

In conclusion, the journey through the pages of this cookbook has been a vibrant exploration of the intersection between health, flavor, and nourishment. By harnessing the power of fresh fruits, vegetables, and herbs, we've embarked on a culinary adventure tailored specifically to support thyroid health and overall well-being.

As you've discovered, juicing offers a delightful way to incorporate a wealth of nutrients into your diet, providing vital support for optimal thyroid function. From energizing morning blends to refreshing citrus elixirs and nutrient-packed vegetable combos, each recipe has been crafted with care to deliver a delicious symphony of flavors and health benefits.

But beyond the juicing recipes themselves, this cookbook serves as a gateway to a lifestyle of vitality and wellness. It's a reminder that nourishing your body with wholesome ingredients is not only beneficial but also a joyous celebration of self-care.

As you embark on your juicing journey, may you savor every sip, delight in every flavor, and revel in the nourishment that these recipes provide. Here's to your continued health, vitality, and the boundless possibilities that await you on your path to thyroid wellness.

www.ingramcontent.com/pod-product-compliance
Lightning Source LLC
Chambersburg PA
CBHW050846260726
48660CB00006B/2478